I0447999

EROTIKA HOT STORIES - Part 4:

Pink Stockings

for men

and

for passionate women

by

Diane Rausch

EROTIKA HOT STORIES - PART 4:
Overwhelmed with Passionate Desires

Stories

Pink Stockings

I am sitting at my home desk and I am wearing pink and black lingerie. It is a pink bra with the contouring black narrow fine lace. My size is 36 C. Lately, C has become a bit small to me, so I started buying 36D. I already told you that my breasts are the perfect size that fits in a man's hand: they are not small, and they are not overly huge. They look kind of big when I am dressed because my waist is small. When I am undressed my breasts are round and perfect, with pink small tender nipples.

I love it when you are squeezing tenderly my breasts. I am also wearing now thin silky stockings that are covering the leg, leaving open about 10 inches of the leg on the top showing a slightly tanned smooth skin. Did I tell you that my skin is very smooth? It's beautiful for the eye and it is absolutely pleasant for the touch.

I love garter belts. I have them in many different colors. It is so exciting to put on sexy lingerie. It is the same excitement as what a man, a hunter, feels when he dresses up for hunting, putting on all the manly clothes, and ammunition. Only a man feels adrenaline rush before the fun of the hunt. The woman feels excitement before giving herself as a trophy to a man. A beautifully packed trophy, a live present.

Men are such sweet creatures. They are never tired

to play games like little boys. Only, when they are adult, they play games with death. I love pilots, because they always risk their lives.

Did I tell you I once loved a young pilot? He was a cute 26-year-old man, and I was a bit older. He had blue eyes, there was usually a smile on his handsome face, and he always wanted sex. I did too.

We were always laughing with him when we would meet for a date. I remember once he said, "Why is it all the time when we meet with you, we always drink alcohol?" And we were laughing. This is what we always did when we met with him: we drank some alcohol, shared latest news, exchanged latest jokes, and then we had sex. I think we drank alcohol because it helped us relax better, and it also gave us some excuse to spend a little time without sex, while we were sharing. Besides, everybody around us did the same. It was the way to behave when you go out.

It was just a customary tribute to a social decency

while in fact we could not look at each other without thinking about sex. Is it how normally the young attractive species of male and female would behave?

It was fun too. I remember I fell in love with him. That's true, that I fell in love with everybody who was handsome or cute or smart or outgoing, or all of this together. Well, this pilot wanted sex a lot. I did too. So we would meet with him and find the place where we could have sex. Did I tell he had beautiful blue eyes, always smiling? He spoke pronouncing "r" sound in a very special way. I loved that about him! Every time, when he called on the phone, I was listening to that cute "r", and I wanted to have him close so much! Now, I have on my CD a man-singer and he pronounces "r" the same way. He even has the pitch of voice as soft as that young pilot used to have. So, I am driving the car, and I am getting so excited when that singer is singing. The pilot could play the guitar and sing. So I would feel as if I am going to the date with the young pilot.

We always fucked like crazy with him. We both loved it. We seemed to never have had enough of it.

Once, he was sent by his work for a long-term business assignment to the city, where women were in the majority of the local population. I remember that we had not seen each other for quite a while, maybe for nine months or so.

Then he came back to the city I lived in. We met. I was up to a big surprise! I remembered from nine months ago him having a certain size of cock, kind of medium size. A good medium size. Now, after working and living in the city where hungry women wanted to have a young handsome good-natured blue-eyed pilot, believe it or not, I knew, I could see and feel, that his cock had grown! It became bigger in size because of the constant use! I do not remember now did I tell him about this observation of mine then, or not.

I know, we were shy. We liked each other, but yet we were shy. There is more excitement when people are shy, and when the element of some kind of mystery remains between a man and a woman who love to fuck each other.

This is the problem with many married couples: the element of mystery gradually disappears, and two people are becoming absolutely bored with each other, and with the same procedures of intimacy they always have. Therefore, a husband and wife have to give each other space. They have to go to different rooms for hours without disturbing each other so they would have this sparkle of joy and missing each other, when they meet in a few hours in a common room, or in the bedroom.

Did I step aside from my initial lingerie wearing? Yes, I did. But this pilot was lately sitting in my head, whenever I listened in my car a similar voice, similar accent, so I had to share the piece about him.

I remember once I saw him when I was flying to London or to Paris. He was working on that airline. Did we speak or not? I think we said "Hello" to each other. How sorry we sometimes feel when we remember old friends who we lost forever. Just the roads of life went totally different directions and we have lost them. I remember once in a while my old friends. Some of them were friends, some of them were lovers. Yet others were friends and lovers. It happened too, more seldom.

OK. That's enough of friends' memories. Let's come back to our black garter belt.

I am wearing light pink very thin silky stockings and a black garter belt. On the top of the garter belt and the stockings I am wearing small pink bikinis with black lace. What a cute, cute look!

I absolutely love lingerie, and I am getting excited over it. Yes, did I tell you that the pilot fucked me so good on the top, and from behind? He was a jolly, sincere, very passionate young man. He loved to fuck. I did too. We loved doing it. He would lick me until I finish, and then he would fuck me until I was exhausted.

The men I was with always knew their routine. They would lick me until I could finish, and then they would fuck me until I was exhausted and completely satisfied.

Now I am sitting here, and I am going to fuck myself. Since I do not have here handy any pilot, and my partner is busy. I am going to fuck myself, and you are going to join me in this act of pleasure.

I am inviting you to join me and get carried away by the flow of the fantasy and pleasure. What is our life? It is a moment of pleasure we live in now. Yesterday already passed. Tomorrow - who knows what tomorrow can bring. We are living the best at this moment! Sexual fantasy is a safe and fun way to take off the tension, and spend a few minutes in a pleasurable and exciting activity.

I love to fuck myself. I love to fuck men different ways, but I love to fuck myself too. I can fuck myself in front of a man, and the appreciative partner would love to watch that.

Ok. Let's see what we have here. We have everything ready to go. I am spreading my legs. I am sitting on a bright pink soft towel, since my computer chair is leather, and I don't want to spot the black leather with my fuck.

My nails are light pink color, nice, smooth and shiny.

I am licking the fingers of my hand and I am going inside my pink bikinis for the delicious tunnel of paradise. It is covered with two lips that are slightly of different size. One is a little smaller, Another one is a little bigger. They are opening like petals of a flower. I am slipping my wet finger between the petals of the pink flower. I am getting wetter and wetter. I rub myself on the lips, around, and occasionally I would go inside the tight tunnel.

Everything around is slippery. I want to get rid of

this bikinis, because they are getting wet. I am taking them off. I love to spread my legs wide and nice. I am so wet. I fondle myself faster and faster, always with the same monotonous movements. I imagine women licking each other. I do not want to lick a woman, but I am turned on by that. So I call for the image in my imagination. That licking image now is joining together with my physical sensations of pleasure from my own wet pink pussy. I am so wet, that it starts making like splashing sounds, because I am doing myself faster and faster. I am fondling myself inside the pussy, the lips are delicious and puffy, they are full of anticipation of the orgasm. I am closing my eyes and I am saying to my imaginable partner, or to you, who is reading my fantasy, "Oh, lick me good, lick me delicious, I want to finish so much. I like to spread my legs for you. I love it when you are licking me. I want you to lick me forever, for hours. Some moments I think I want licking to last forever, yet at the other moments I think that I want to have a strong orgasm. I want to explode good and sweet.

I am fucking myself with my hand, faster and faster, I am moving on a chair. I am thinking about open wide legs and pink pussy. I love tender licking with the tense tongue. Now the tongue goes around clit, it is sucking it very tenderly. Not too much. In reality. I am doing my clit with my finger, that is very wet. Only wet can be pleasant. Wet finger is like a tongue.

I am rubbing my clit and then I go inside the tunnel. Now I am thinking that the tongue is licking my clit, and the man's hot and tense and tight and hard cock is going inside my pussy - simultaneously. Oh, how I love that cute cock, and I whisper with a lust, "More, more my baby, do me simultaneously - in the clit with the tongue, and in the pussy with your hard hot cock. I will finish soon. It is coming. Faster, faster. Oh, how good you are sucking my clitoris, and how good is your thick pink cock going fast into my pussy.

Oh, I am finishing, I am climaxing now, lick me, lick me, you have to lick me until I finish my orgasm otherwise it will not feel complete. Yes, yes, how good! I am finishing so strongly, and it is lasting so many seconds. I am in the skies of pleasure, the highest pleasure! I am releasing the portion of my sperm. My towel is very wet.

What a relief! Next time I am with a man, I want to be fucked right after the climax. It is the beautiful feeling - to be fucked right after the climax. It feels like you are continuing finishing for the next few minutes. The cock goes directly into open bottom of my pussy. Everything open and orgasmic, after the orgasm. Everything in my pussy remembers the seconds of heavenly incomparable pleasure.

Oh, thank you, thank you, my darling for sharing with me my beautiful moments of pleasure! I can relax now and watch TV or read a book.

I Am Not A Man (About My Dream Woman)

This story is an aesthetic excursion into the woman's mind. Men! Do not be offended! Even if you recognize yourself in some of my sketches, relax, and think, that it is not you, but your neighbor that you do not like too much. I am just having here a general talk, so do not feel too personal. But, you will benefit from this voyage - you will know next time better something what is not usually talked about or discussed. You will have these inner basics of sexual and gender-related behavioral intuition. So, relax, and get informed. In the end of the chapter I'll sex you up to relax you and cheer you up.

Although I am not a man, I want to describe my feelings that I think I would have towards women if I were a man. Why do I want to do it? Because there are so many attractive women around, so sometimes you can't help it, thinking, "I wonder, if I were a man, would I want to fuck this woman or not?"

My next thought about being a man and asking myself about wanting a particular woman comes to, "Well, if I were a man, I would probably want to fuck everything that moves, like any regular man." Generally speaking, it seems true, at the first approach to the topic, or, for some, so to say, "emergency-fuck" life situations, such as drunkenness, feeling of a herd, brethren, of a company, brotherhood, extreme sexual hunger, etc. However, if to take the second look at this matter, and analyze the psychology between men and women, I would probably be inclined to have the type of a woman of my preference and liking instead of disorderly chasing all the cute skirts.

You will also see what I know that you might have not known just for the reason because I am a woman and I am a different person with different experiences, urges, and outlooks!

I want to touch here a topic of prostitutes since it is an ancient sex trade in our world. There is no man, and no woman, who hasn't thought about their attitude to the most ancient profession, or who doesn't have a certain standing towards it. This is why I want to say a few words here about it.

This chapter of the book is not a mere sex-pleasure-arousing tool; it is also a thought-evoking instrument.

That's how a person is different from an animal - we can think!, and learn to enjoy the direction of our brain-work to our health benefit, our psychological balance, and aesthetic contentment of mind.

There is a topic that I have not been able to share with many people for this or that reason, the name of which is chiefly "expecting being misunderstood". The pages of this chapter are an appropriate pasture for feeding these kinds of thoughts in the freedom of fresh air and absence of hostile intellectual winds.

So, in terms of the topic about the prostitutes, there is a category of men who, when asked about their attitude to prostitutes, would say, "I never would pay for sex". I'll tell you, category "Mr No Pay". The first life observation is that you are probably simply greedy. In addition, you are most likely "narcissistic without grounds", and have something wrong with your self-esteem feeling.

Greediness. Before I touch this low and pathetic

topic, I want to remind of something to the men, who are reading these pages, in case they have never known this before. You know, what is the most repulsive, disgusting and ridiculous for a woman? You thought it was a small penis? No! Nobody cares about the penis in the long run.

A greedy man is the most repulsive for a woman! Now, after this knowledge, those, who can admit to yourselves, in the quiet of your privacy, that you possess this unattractive quality, do not look for other excuses. It's fruitless. A woman knows a greedy type of man. She ridicules him. Just try to learn how to be more generous. Women love generous men. Do not flatter yourself, that your beautiful smile or eyes would attract them. Your generosity will do, for sure. Now, I am not going here into the topic of gigolos and their living on the expense of older rich women. Gigolos love themselves and do not have a better profession or any skills, neither dignity. The older women, who have lust for younger man, will pay you, as the older men pay to younger women. There's no difference.

Nevertheless, here I am talking about regular layers of society, leaving these gigolo-things and misalliances alone.

The greediness or stinginess is a strong and overpowering feeling that people might have from their parents, from their other upbringing conditions or surroundings. Greediness is not always connected to poverty. Some men of modest means can be very generous, and yet, a man from a rich family can be very greedy. How do I know? From experience!

I was dating once a rich and stingy man. His biggest fear was to be discovered by other people that he was greedy like hell. So, in public places, like dancing bars, he would buy cocktails to everybody so that everybody would say, "Jack is the most generous and the nicest person I know". However, I knew Jack as his girlfriend of 14 months. He was the stingiest guy, he was revoltingly stingy. But I soon figured out it was a mental disease, so I then thought of him as of a mentally sick person. Which was a true approach and assessment. This kind of man is mentally-socially disabled: while worrying about other people's opinions this kind would show all the greediness to the closest person.

The man was very well-educated. He did not date market-women. So he knew that I would never go around and start bad-mouthing him. Any other decent well-mannered woman (believe it or not - it often directly correlates with education) - we are not capable of these methods. So, the guy was protected of ill fame this way.

So, the first motive of "I would never pay a prostitute" is sheer greediness. The second motive, as I mentioned earlier, is the wrong perception of your own self-esteem. If you are a man, you are paying to the woman not because you cannot get women for free, but because Number One - you can pay (literally:

you have money after your bills paid), and Number Two - you want this particular woman's body no matter who she is.

You know, I noticed that the unpleasant type would say, "I would never pay...", reaffirming their unpleasantness. The regular type would just keep silent about the topic, since there is nothing particularly good or deserving to brag about, if you are older than 14 years old.

I believe, there is one more kind of men, who are not greedy to pay a prostitute, and have everything intact with their identity and self-esteem, but just simply do not respect the type of women represented by the profession of prostitute. I respect this type of men, because they are honest. They just do not want to deal with a woman who is passing armies between her legs or by her mouth. It is a feeling of not accepting the filth. I do understand that.

As for the "Mr Hurt Self-Esteem", I'd say, "Come from the Skies of your Self-Esteem that nobody is interested in, since people are sincerely interested only in nice qualities; so, come from your cloud, land yourself on the sinful earth, look around. There are famous people, celebrities who love to use prostitutes. Do you think they cannot have anybody for free or for the signature on a postcard? Sure they do. They have infinite choice of fresh and young women at any time; the women, who would be happy and grateful, and remember their sin all the rest of their lives. So, stop pretending, and look at yourself in the mirror".

The world would be a much better place without greedy people, especially men. When a woman is greedy, she is a woman. She has her reasons. There are no reasons for a greedy man. A man is a bread-winner, a strong, smart, and able. One of his "manliness" traits is to have a profession that will put a roof above his head and secure a woman near him, because he has that roof, and he knows how to pay his bills. A woman is an obedient, soft creature. I am not talking here about upside-down values, and all directions-variations of the modern society.

I am coming back to my initial topic of conversation: if I were a man. I warned you, the greediness is a powerful feeling; now you see for yourselves how far away from the topic it threw me!

If I were a man, I would have any woman I want to have. If I happened to be in the mood to have that prostitute that I thought I liked, I would have her. I don't think I would be the frequenter of a bordello, but I would certainly try "young and free-expressing". With precautions of getting some disease, of course.

Prostitutes can be of different kinds. Some are just going through the period of life when they cannot get enough of sex, so they think, "Why I just make some money on the way of my ongoing insatiable hunger for sex, since my father and uncle are not rich, and if to think about it, I have never had neither of the two!". Some prostitutes may be of regular families. Others maybe of poor families, or of broken families. All prostitutes have their reasons. And yes, this is their conscious choice of a life-style, no matter if they say, "I need to get my child through schooling". The latter is the most ridiculous statement: to earn for good cause by prostitution? Excuses, excuses! It is an old practice with women to show themselves off in a better light than they actually are existing. Keeping up with the Joneses! (almost, since prostitution has fallen out even off Joneses)

And Men, who are reading my entertaining stories, just be aware, that many women are not proud of what they had done in their young years, and you will never know the underwater side of the iceberg of your wife, girlfriend, neighbor, or colleague, after they cross the line of forty, or got married, or whatever their crossing line was. So sleep peacefully in your happy ignorance.

Of course, there are some women who are naturally honest and never been around many men. This kind was bound to their family obligations exercising self-control beyond self-freedom, and they often times are naturally frigid too. I don't think it is a big heroic deed to be an honest woman if you do not like sex and frigid. And I am deeply respectful and feel sorry for those women, who had to suffer in honesty, neglecting their inside fire of passions, for example, because they having gotten married at an early age. We all have our own destiny that we sometimes can slightly control, if we are somewhat lucky. Our lives are full or relativity and circumstantiation.

I once had a friend who was telling about his acquaintance Bill, who did not like sex. So, Bill had the same not-loving-sex kind of a girlfriend. They would come to a weekend-getaway hotel, sit on the wide bed, eat pizza, drink sodas and watch TV. Their minds would get never crossed by the thought of enjoying sex. What a waste of time and location for many people!

If I were a man, I would love a woman who is smart, but who has enough tact not to show the incidents when she is smarter than me. A woman should be always respectful of man's dignity.

I would love an average height, not too tall (giant height reminds me of big funny robots; maybe it is good on the podium, who knows; in real life there are not too many people who are over 6 or 7 feet, so these towering women look out of place unless it is the site of giants or dwarfs - the other extreme).

I would love a woman of 5.6 (about 167cm).   On the heels she is rather tall. Without the heels she is average.

I love her to have a womanly body with no-showing muscle shapes. I am not fascinated with athletes in a regular life. Well, of course, I would not mind to sleep with an athlete, why not, out of curiosity, but I think, frankly, that they are boring people, overwhelmed with their keeping in shape and their narrow kind of sports.

Sometimes I read that they are many-sided and educated. Well, let's say, I don't buy it too much. There are always exceptions to the rules though.

I would like a woman with a good figure. Now let's comment here on a woman's figure. I see, that many people are mislead with a shapely waste ignoring the shortness of legs. People! Open your eyes! Short legs are ugly, whatever narrow her waste is.

No, please don't give me short legs, and don't give me the waste line that starts at the thighs. You know, there's a type of a long waste, and then suddenly a bubble, where are thighs supposed to be.

No bubbles please. Look at the classical pictures and figures. The line of a hip should be round starting a bit lower than a waist. The buttocks and "poppy" should be perfect size. We don't like wide-hipped "cortitas" (short-things).

If I were a man, give me a woman, who goes and I can't believe how beautiful is her shape.

I would seduce the woman I like, at any price. Well, reasonable price. I am not going to go after somebody's wife, or after a stubborn babe. I don't like them stubborn. If I were a man, the woman of my dreams is not stubborn. She knows romance, and she likes to be romanced. She like jokes and fun, and I would joke with her and have fun.

Then I'll get her to bed. In the bed, I will lick her until she is done, or the way she wants it. Men! Do not lick your women until they cannot tell the difference between tongue and not tongue. Do not lick them too much. I've been there. It is very weird: when you don't have it, you think you can have it endlessly, and yet, when you have it endlessly, you wish you could have it in moderation, so you could preserve your desires. Men! Do not kill your woman's desires and passions by overlicking her. No matter how much you like it. Go and quietly lick something else (of course, I mean somebody! LOL) to satisfy your licking urges. If you overlick your woman, she will get frozen, and it will be hard for her to want sex anymore.

You want to keep her interested. Adjust to her speed. I know there is a big problem in the world of romance and marriages: the problem of inequality of a sexual drive in 2 partners. Well, being one of the partners, learn your second half, and try to get used to their desires. In the first weeks or a couple of months, I think you should know, that this partner is for you or not for you. Then you have to make that decision - to stay with them or to leave.

I've had everything - regular satisfaction, regular dissatisfaction, and over sexing to the point when you are not happy because you know you lost your sex drive for the reason of the over-zealousness in sex from your second half.

I wish everybody to find your perfect partner, rather to find your perfect balance in self-sexing - with your partner, and without him or her.

And now, for men, I will give you an oral delicious session.

And for men and women, I will do myself.

Let's relax, my captain.

Look at me. How beautiful are your eyes, and your face features.

I love your eyes and your face features. I love your little habits when you speak, when you smoke a joint, when you are sitting calmly and business-like trying to do your job.

I am sneaking to you and starting fondling your jeans. Something that is inside. It grows. I like how it grows. It is like a little animal. It has life of its own. It is becoming big and warm. It is becoming almost hot, and it wants to get out of the jeans.

I am unzipping your jeans, and taking my cute animal out of the pants. It's the cutest little animal! It has a head, and the eyes, like those of a big dragon-fly, and it has a mouth. It looks a little silly, with a head and big eyes-cheeks of a dragon fly. But it is the cutest thing! I am kissing it, and kissing it, and I am taking it into my mouth. I am sliding it slowly inside. I am sliding it inside to my throat, to the point when it touches the back of my mouth. Then I go in and out, in and out. It is slippery and it goes nice and easy. Nice and easy.

Then I take it out and I kiss it on the top along the length of the animal. I kiss it into the slippery skin. Then I lick it, and I take it back into the mouth.

You are doing me into the mouth. Faster and faster.

Explode! I am ready to swallow all your sperm deep into my throat.

Doing Myself with the Water: A True Story

Once upon a time there was a waiter in a big international hotel who liked me a lot. The hotel was the biggest and the most popular in a port capital city. It was an interesting place to have a good time, since it had always interesting tourists and foreigners of all kinds. The waiter's name was Joshua. He worked in a big restaurant, where I liked to go at that time. It was difficult to get there, but Joshua could always find for me a table of some back up reservations. Joshua was patently waiting for me to complete all my entertaining activities. He was waiting for the deep dark night when I would join him, once in a while, visiting his home. He looked like a typical waiter, and I did not like his looks. Blondish, serviceable. However, he was very kind and he liked me with all his servant's heart. Besides, the cuisine in the restaurant was very good, and Joshua would fulfill all my gastronomic wishes. For this reason I felt that I wanted to reward him once in a while to keep him content. I knew he was suffering when he watched me go with somebody other.

Joshua's Reward

I went into his bathtub. We made the water pleasantly warm temperature. I was lying on the bottom of the bathtub with my legs wide apart and up. Nice long legs. Spread wide, up, and apart. Beautiful!

Joshua would sit near the bathroom on a low stool and watch me like a hungry eagle. An eagle hungry for the sight. He was eagerly devouring with his eyes my sexual act with myself.

I would be directing the water (not too strong and not too weak) onto my open pussy. My beautiful open pink pussy. My eyes are closed. I am in a feast of emotions. Gentle, gentle, stronger, and stronger. The water can be better than a man-lover with it monotonous flow. A man-lover can get tired, and thus get out of rhythm, but the water can't. So it goes monotonously on my sweat pussy lips, on my pink clit, interchangeably, here, and there, and overwhelmingly pleasant feeling of lust, desire, ecstasy is possessing now my mind, and body, and pussy. I am starting groaning of pleasure. More, more, more... I am moving my hips in tact with my coming orgasm. With my mind I know that Joshua is all overwhelmed with a pleasurable watching experience, too. I am happy that I can make him happy at least once in a while for all his loyalty to me. I try to relax and be absolutely free, without thinking that somebody is watching me. Now I belong to myself, and my orgasmic experiences.

Harder, harder, faster, faster, more intensive, I am coming, exploding, I am moaning loud to relieve myself of the coming orgasm.

O-o-o-oh, what an amazing fuck!

My "sperm" is all washed and my pussy is pacified with the running water.

What a pleasure!

Everybody is happy, Joshua, and I. The act of pleasure has been accomplished to our both satisfaction.